Open in the Front

Don't Forget to Laugh

Aimee Kintzel

Prologue

Ladies ~ Get your girls checked!

Gentlemen ~ Yes, you can get breast cancer. Watch for lumps. Men don't get mammograms, so be vigilant. If you find something suspicious, see your doctor. If this makes you uncomfortable, find a cute female doctor and make it an adventure.

I get my mammogram every year. It is for this reason my cancer was found early and was completely curable. I know it's not fun and especially sucks for us vertically challenged gals, but it saved my life. Because my cancer was found early, I have had a relatively easy journey. Cancer sucks, but it doesn't have to consume you.

Cancer is a scary word! Being told you have cancer is even scarier. This book is being written to remind you that even though you have cancer, you can still have fun and laugh. We found so many things humorous. At times that felt completely wrong, and that is fine. This was my journey. Another person can travel in whatever vehicle they want. I chose humor. Don't let the doom of the word cancer consume you. I truly believe that one's attitude and outlook is half the battle when dealing with life events.

I did not do any research except when I really wanted to understand something at the moment. I am not going to throw a lot of facts and figures at you. I find If I dwell on those things, it can bring me down. Sometimes, I find that a little knowledge can be dangerous, especially to my psyche.

Most importantly, this is not a gimmick to advocate for my doctors and hospitals. I will be happy to recommend them if asked, though. I believe I had the best.

I am simply going to tell you my story.

Contents

Chapter 1
Boob Squoosh Boogie

I try to schedule my annual tests for the months surrounding my birthday at the end of July. With that being said, my mammogram was scheduled for June 26, 2024, and my colonoscopy was scheduled for August 2. I had already had my full-body skin check a few months earlier. I was checking things off my list.

June 26 was just like any other day. As I sat in the waiting room of the hospital, I saw someone I knew. We chatted about why each of us was there. I told her I was there for my "boob squoosh boogie." We laughed. She was going to be having hip surgery and was there for a test to make sure she would be able to have it on the scheduled date. I was called back. She wished me good luck, as I did her, and off I went.

The mammogram technician, also known as mammograph or mammography technologist, was so gentle and kind. She took me to the mammography suite, where I changed into my stylish hospital gown (I would become very familiar with these gowns) to wait. There was a TV in the waiting area, and I was offered something to drink. The wait was short.

We entered the mammogram room and went to work. We made small talk. I joked about my height. I am short which makes the mammogram just a touch more challenging. We did our best to make an uncomfortable situation bearable. I wondered silently, "Does playing with my boobs make her as uncomfortable as it does me?" We got the job done. She sent me on my way with the standard, "We will contact you if we find something." I have been getting my mammograms for many years, and I had never gotten that follow-up call.

Imagine my surprise when I got a MyChart message from the hospital stating they had found something suspicious on my mammogram. I go every year. I've never had anything suspicious. It was not alarming. It was a blurry spot, and the doctor just wanted to look at it a little closer. They didn't say as much, but I interpreted he didn't really think it was anything to be concerned about at that point. On July 11, 2024, back to the mammography technician I went for an ultrasound of my left breast. She sent it off to the radiologist, who looked at the report while we waited. He determined he would like to look at another spot as well, so we went back to the ultrasound machine. She sent the images off to the radiologist, who called once he had had a chance to look at them. He said a lot of words. I heard a few. Two spots, 11 millimeters, biopsy. Biopsy. BIOPSY! I was not alarmed or worried, but I felt a surreal numbness that is really hard to explain. I walked out of the hospital on autopilot. I smiled at the people I passed by and did my best to pretend I was not just told I might have cancer.

That night, while sharing space in the bathroom (we've been married for over 30 years; there are not a lot of secrets here), I told my husband, my sweet, tenderhearted husband, that I had to have a biopsy. He immediately started to cry. He didn't want me to have to go through this. We have watched both of our mothers deal with breast cancer. His mother had both breasts removed, radiation, and chemotherapy. She lost her hair and her fingernails. She survived. My mom had a lumpectomy, chemotherapy, and radiation. I don't remember her losing her hair or fingernails. But different cancers equate to different treatments. She survived. Jim didn't want me to have to go through any of that. I told him I was not worried or scared but that we knew I would eventually face some form of cancer. We just didn't know when or what kind (more on that later). This would not be my first biopsy either. In early 2013, during a routine blood workup, we found that my white blood cell count was high. I had no other symptoms, but since my mom had a form of leukemia, the oncologist wanted to do a bone marrow biopsy. I was terrified at that time. I have heard so many horror stories about the bone marrow biopsy. It really was a piece of cake. They numb you and place a large needle or catheter into the bone of your hip to collect marrow from inside it. It did not hurt, except for the cramp I got in my butt from trying to lie still. The doctor did not find that amusing. I don't think he understood my joke. At any rate, the result came out negative for any of the things they were looking for. I have also had a skin lesion removed and biopsied. Again, it came back negative for cancer.

The night I told Jim I would need to have a breast biopsy, there was a lot of hugging. He's a hugger, always has been. My grandmother used to say, "You haven't been hugged until you've been hugged by Jim Kintzel." I don't usually get those hugs. His hands wander to different places when he hugs me. I got those hugs that night.

I still had not told anybody else what was going on. I told Jim I did not want to tell anybody anything… yet. I told him he could choose somebody he trusted if he felt like he needed to talk to somebody, but I did not want a lot of people to know anything at this point. It was nobody's business. We didn't know what the outcome would be or what would happen next. Nobody needed to know. I told my friend Betsy, who works with Jim because I thought she might be someone he would choose to talk to. Betsy has been a friend to both of us for many years. She grew up in the same general area as Jim and has known him since childhood. I became friends with her sister in high school, but we drifted apart over the years. Betsy has been steady. I even sent my daughter, Erin, off to a concert with her when Jim and I couldn't attend. She calls Erin Baby Girl, like I do. I knew I could trust her to keep this information in her pocket until I was ready to share it.

Chapter 2
Biopsy to Diagnosis

A biopsy was scheduled for July 25, 2024. Thus far, the only person I had told anything to was my boss, and only because I would have to ask for time off for all of these damn tests. I am not one to miss work, and I feel extremely guilty whenever I do. I swear I should have been Catholic because everything makes me feel guilty, and boy, was I about to feel it.

I planned to take myself for the biopsy in Fort Wayne, an hour's drive. It was only a biopsy; I would be able to drive, and I wouldn't have any results that day to make me emotional. My amazing support system felt differently. Jim was going to let me go because I insisted I could do this on my own and it's just easier, sometimes, to roll your eyes and walk away without arguing with me. However, Betsy refused to let me go alone and said she would take me. When I told Jim this, he said he agreed that he didn't want me going alone. I think I might have even heard a sigh of relief. So, it was settled that Betsy would drive me to Fort Wayne.

On July 25, I drove to Jim and Betsy's workplace (hers and our son also worked there). Betsy drove me to Fort Wayne from there. Boy, did we raise eyebrows. Everybody thought they needed to know where we were going and what was going on. Betsy's son actually tracked her location by GPS on her phone and had figured out where we were and began texting her in a panic, thinking she was the one we were there for. So Betsy had to tell him what was going on. I'm learning you can't keep this shit secret for very long. He promised not to tell my son, Chad.

Everyone at the Cancer Center was incredible, from the check-in receptionist to the radiology nurse, who included Betsy in explaining what would be happening, to the ultrasound tech and radiologist. Each of them did whatever they could to make me feel comfortable. I couldn't have asked for a better experience. A plus, was that they only found the one spot from the ultrasound when they did their ultrasound to locate where to pull tissue from. Therefore, they only needed to biopsy one spot plus lymph nodes. The radiologist was phenomenal. He made light conversation. We talked about our kids and grandkids and what kind of books we like to read. As it turned out, we enjoyed some of the same authors. James Patterson was a favorite of both of us. The technicians held my hands and patted my leg when they thought I was in pain. They could not have made the experience any easier. When it was done, I was given an ice pack and told I could do normal activities with the exception of swimming and bathing for 48 hours.

I had previously planned a weekend getaway at a casino hotel in Michigan City, Indiana, for the next day. I had received a complimentary (yea I know, I've paid for it many times over) weekend at the Blue Chip Casino and Spa. My travel partner/partner in crime, Angela would be going with me. Angela is one of those friends who comes into your life out of nowhere, but it seems like you've known them forever. I know that we met through our children, who were in 4-H together, but I can't begin to tell you when or how our friendship bloomed. She has become my ride-or-die for sure. If ever I need someone to tag along with me, I know she will if she's available. We have sat and cried with one another through hurting children, health scares, and stress. I can tell you unequivocally that I would not have survived some of my life trials without her. We both have husbands who would prefer to stay home than go on adventures, so we adventure together. We like to tell people that we are the other's devil on their shoulder. I only smoke when I am with her, and she only drinks when she is with me. On the way, we stopped at a rest stop, and I bought a pack of cigarettes. I only smoke when I'm stressed… or drunk. I lit a cigarette and jumped in, and we got back on the road. A few miles down the road, I just blurted it out. I told her I had had a biopsy the day before, why Betsy had taken me, and why I had not asked her to take me. I told her I was fine and did not hurt but that I wouldn't be able to partake in the swimming pool during our stay. We enjoyed our weekend, gambled, shopped at the outlet mall, ate a lot of good food, drank, and fed the slot machines a lot of money. I need to learn to play the tables.

On July 30, 2024, the day after my birthday, I received a MyChart message. When I opened the app, I found the results of my biopsy: malignant concordant diagnosis of invasive ductal carcinoma. My phone rang while I was looking at those words. It was my primary care doctor with the same news. She was so gentle and told me how sorry she was. She would be putting me on the cancer registry and start making referrals.

Invasive… Carcinoma… More words… These words were terrifying.

Happy Birthday to me!

Chapter 3
Telling My People

I did not want to tell anybody until we had a plan, but Jim insisted I needed to tell the kids NOW. We have two children. Our daughter, Erin, is the older of the two, and our son, Chad, is the younger. They are the lights of my life. I have made it my life mission to make their lives as easy as possible and to always be here for them. I didn't want to tell them... ever. This was the single hardest thing I have done throughout this journey and maybe my entire life. I did not want to do it! Up to this point, I had not actually said the words, "I have cancer." Admitting that I had a monster in my body that would try to kill me and the fact I had no control over what would happen next was unnerving. I wasn't scared. I was never really scared about the diagnosis itself, but saying those words out loud terrified me.

Chad lives with us, so we stopped him on his way in the door from work. After we all looked at one another awkwardly for a beat or two, I blurted out, "I have breast cancer." He was silent for a moment. Like his dad, Chad is a tenderhearted young man of few words. Finally, he gathered himself and said only two words, "How bad?" We told him we didn't know and that we had just received the diagnosis. I explained that it was found by my mammogram and that it hadn't been seen last year, so I was certain I would be fine. He stayed in the room while we called (facetimed) his sister, Erin. Erin is my feisty, mouthy mini-me. We seldom have a conversation where we aren't slamming someone or something. Often, it's each other, always in love. She knew something was up because we don't call out of the blue, especially late in the evening. We text a lot. You will learn most of it is pretty inappropriate, and if people read a lot of what we text to one another, they would probably commit both of us. But that's for another time. She answered very apprehensively and immediately asked what was wrong. Again, I had to blurt it out. It was the only way I could say the words. She started to cry, and I told her I was not scared or worried and told the whole story about how they hadn't seen it last year, so it must be small… I'm gonna be fine. Somewhere during this conversation, Chad excused himself and went downstairs.

Jim sees his parents every day when he stops in after feeding his livestock. So he had that conversation for me. Two people I did not have to tell.

Next was my parents. We tried to visit them every other weekend or so and a visit was due. We sat down and chatted a little bit, and then I finally blurted out again that we had something we needed to tell them. I said the words again, "I have breast cancer." Again, it was quiet for a beat or two then the questions started. They knew the questions since we had been through it with her. We told them we would be going to the oncologist on Monday and would have more information after that. I could tell they were both concerned, but their words were reassuring. We've traveled this path before. (I will talk more about it later, but I have a lot of cancer in my family.) We are strong, and we will beat this. My parents are the best! They wanted to make sure I told my brother so they could feel free to talk about it and not have to worry about giving away anything I hadn't already shared. So I made a point of stopping in to see him one day at lunchtime and told him. I promised to keep him informed.

I decided that this was a private matter and that it would not be broadcast all over social media. You know, you see the people who post about every single thing that is troubling them, "Please pray for me." I have friends I really love, and I will send up a prayer or a smoke signal or whatever, But for the love of God, stop asking for prayers every time you get a fart stuck! Stop airing all your laundry, clean or dirty, on social media. Just STOP! I held to that, and only the people I hold dearest to my heart were told until I was through the storm.

I called and canceled my colonoscopy.

Chapter 4
China Doll

After we told all the pertinent people, I learned that my life would not be the same for a while. I am a very independent person. I don't ask for help. If I want something done, I either do it or try to do it and screw it up so that Jim has to fix it for me. Jim, though tenderhearted and very affectionate, does not baby me. That's just not our relationship. I lift, I carry, I mow, I garden. That all changed in an instant.

Remember my hugs that are just a little different from everyone else's? We have always been a very amorous pair. I won't go into detail about some of our escapades, but this part is important to my story. He always has his hands on my boobs. Always! I believe he has radar when it comes to my boobs. He is like a dog with a cheese wrapper. He can be in another room, and I swear he can hear me take off my bra. This changed the day I got my diagnosis. He was suddenly afraid of my boobs. He didn't come running when I was undressing. He would barely look at them when he caught a glimpse.

My tumor (MY tumor! So possessive) was in my left breast. Jim would continue to fondle my right breast but was terrified of Lefty or Louise, as I came to call her. I would mention this on occasion and tell him that she was feeling neglected. He would say he didn't want to hurt me. I would explain that I had a tumor that I could not feel. I was not sick. I didn't believe he was going to hurt me. But this continued … until it didn't!

Jim started treating me like a China doll. While this was nice, I appreciated how sweet he was. Like I said, this just was not our relationship. He would not let me do anything for myself: lift, carry etc. Between this and his not wanting to touch me, I was about to lose my mind. I was just about at my breaking point. Finally, one beautiful summer day, I was outside playing with our grandson. Bennett has endless amounts of energy and so as I was following him around, I began to sweat, as one does on a hot and sunny summer afternoon. Jim got home from work and, saw that I was sweating, and told me that I needed to go inside. I said, "I am not sick; I don't need to go inside." We argued back and forth. He insisted. At this point, I was over it. I told him, "Fine! But it is too nice for the 4-year-old to be inside, so you are going to have to entertain him." I then went inside and sat my ass in front of the tv and did nothing. I did not fix supper, and neither did I do anything else for the rest of the night. After all, I might break; I am a China doll. I would tell this story many times. Most people laughed, but one person in particular told me that she found this very sweet, as her ex-husband would not have even acknowledged her "illness." She explained that while she was recuperating after their third child, he offered no help whatsoever and expected her to do everything for herself and everybody else. At that moment, I decided to accept the coddling without complaint, and life was good again.

There came a point when Jim would not even look at my chest. You know how a woman will be speaking, and the man is looking at her chest and not her face… and she will point to her face and say, "My eyes are up here."? Well, it got to the point where I would look at him and say, "Hey, my boobs are down here." He began to get a little more comfortable but still would not pay any attention to Louise (Lefty) unless I complained.

Chapter 5

The Journey Begins

The journey began with an appointment in Fort Wayne again on August 5. We would travel to the same facility where the biopsy was performed. Jim and I met with the oncologist. The oncologist was another very kind person. We were given a lot of information. A lot of words were said. Many I didn't know and later looked up. We have all heard the Stage 4 horror stories about cancer. My cancer was Stage 1. This means it was small. We were told that the tumor was approximately 11 mm in size. I measured that and compared it to an M & M.

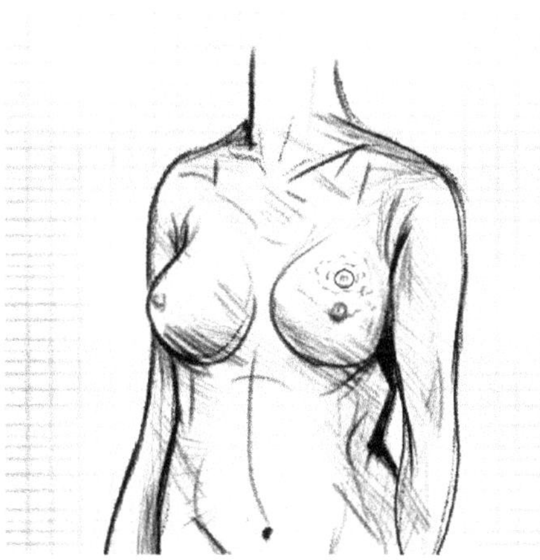

One thing I had not previously heard about or acknowledged was the grading of tumors. My tumor was Grade 1. This means it was slow growing. The doctor explained, so slowly, that it was very likely there the previous year when I had my mammogram, but it was not yet visible. This all sounded like good news. As good as can be for having cancer.

We were also told that this was a hormone-positive tumor. I'm sure you have seen the commercials on TV about HR+, HER2+, positive, negative, etc. My cancer was HR+. This stands for Hormone Receptor Positive. This basically means the estrogen my body is still producing, because I have not completed my amazing trip through menopause, is feeding the tumor. Don't ask me what the HER2+ or all the other positives and negatives are all about. I could have looked it up, but it didn't pertain to me. Unless you are a facts and figures person and not prone to agonizing about your worries, I would recommend that you don't research any more than you need to. What this information meant was that my cancer was hormone-fed, and I would have to take an estrogen blocker for at least 5 years once my treatment was completed. This, she explained, would basically put me into menopause if I wasn't already. I told her I pretty much was already, but she wanted to do a blood test to determine where I was on this path. So, she sent me to the lab in their facility before we left. As it turned out, I was still Perimenopausal. Oh Joy! The hot flashes, night sweats, and mood swings will get worse. Buckle up family.

We were told that we would go for a surgical consult, and it is likely that I would have radiation after surgery and then possibly chemotherapy, depending on the Oncotype test score. One of those words I had to look up. It is a screening of the genetic make-up of the tumor that is completed once the tumor is removed. If the score is too high, it might be likely to recur, so chemotherapy would be ordered.

I was presented with a tote bag full of goodies. There was a portfolio notebook with brochures and information about the care team at the hospital. I thought I would be using this thing all the time. I didn't. I am a paper person, and I like to write everything down. In the beginning, I did just that. As time went on I wrote down less and less until I stopped writing anything except appointments in my calendar.

The next step was to schedule an appointment with a breast surgeon. While Parkview has a breast surgeon on staff at the Fort Wayne campus, she was booked solid until the end of the month, and I wouldn't even be able to get an appointment for a consultation until then. When you're faced with these uncertainties, waiting is not ideal, especially when you are impatient like me. They told us that they have some surgeons that they often work with. There was one at another hospital in Fort Wayne, one in Carmel, Indiana and that there was one in particular that people really seemed to like who was located in Anderson, Indiana. A two-hour drive from our home. They had just scheduled someone else with her for the following week. Without hesitating or even consulting with Jim, I said, let's try it. They were able to schedule a consultation appointment with her for the very next day. Heck yah! Let's get this train moving!

The doctor wanted to do a breast exam before we left that day, and so the disrobings began. She left the room while I got into the robe (open in the front). Mr. Boob Man got excited at getting to watch me unclothe without trying to hide from him. So, I shook them in front of him. This became a thing. We tried to have fun at every scary appointment. The doctor came back in and did the exam. Nothing special. My tumor was small, and you could not feel it. Jim watched patiently as someone else fondled my breasts.

Chapter 6

Next Stop, Breast Surgeon

The next day, we plugged the address into the GPS and headed South. The trip was uneventful but scenic, as the GPS took us through the countryside. Jim liked this because there was no traffic to deal with. We found the hospital without any trouble, but what door do we go in? We sat in the car and argued about what to do. Finally, I got out of the car and started toward a door with my handy, dandy new tote bag full of goodies over my shoulder. We were early and the office was dark when we arrived. I began to panic that we had gone to the wrong place. Then someone spotted us and opened the door. They had been at lunch.

After a short wait, we were taken to an examination room. I was given a robe and told to strip from the waist up and put on the robe (open in front). Here we go again. Jim got excited. We had a rather long wait in the exam room, approximately an hour. Some folks would have been angry at the wait. We were feeling the go-with-the-flow vibe already and did our best to be patient. After a two-hour drive, you don't want to be there for just 5 minutes anyway.

When she finally came in, my surgeon was still wearing scrubs. She was a lovely young lady. She had long brunette hair, a beautiful face, and kind eyes. What does brunette hair and a beautiful face have to do with anything? Nothing, but these are the things that caught my attention. And as such, I have dubbed her, Dr. Beauty. Dr. Beauty apologized again and again. She stated that she had been with a patient who was getting her drain tubes removed (more on those later), and she had brought her daughter with her. She said the daughter had a lot of questions. I told her she could stop right there. She had just told me everything I needed to know about herself and confirmed to me that I was in the right place. While I may have had to wait on her, this told me she would spend as much time with ME as I needed. Not only was MY breast surgeon kind and patient, but she was also very knowledgeable. She said a lot more words. But even though many of them were still foreign to us, she made them make sense. I felt like I was home. We talked about my case and the options I would be facing. I have always said if I ever get this diagnosis, I would just “hack ‘em off.” Watching our mothers deal with it and knowing the likelihood that our daughter might one day face it had sealed this in my brain. I told the surgeon this and that I was ok with that. They are just fat bags, and since I am not having any more kids, I don’t need them for anything. I looked over at Jim and added, “Except for him.” I wanted to be the example Erin or anyone else who may have to face this disease, needed to help them make this decision. I have never wavered on this.

The surgeon did another breast exam, and then she used the ultrasound machine to pinpoint where everything was. She found only the original 11 mm spot on my left breast and nothing on the right. She wanted to place markers to make sure that they took only what they needed to. I think she thought I was joking about hacking those puppies off. I wasn't! She wanted me to do another test to make sure everything was in order before she scheduled marker placement and surgery. She wanted me to go for a breast MRI. This would show if there were any outlier cells that weren't being seen by ultrasound. Again, nothing close to our home offered this, so I would travel to Kokomo, Indiana. An easy drive but yet another 1-hour long trip.

We also talked about genetic testing, as I have a long family history of cancer, including my mom's breast cancer and my dad's colon cancer. The nurse navigator communicated with my oncologist's office, and everyone agreed that genetic testing should be done. Blood was drawn that day. I should probably mention that I have thin, fickle veins that do not like to share. I would tell each person that I would be their challenge for the day and tell them to go to the top of my hand. Nobody really likes to do this, but I know that one bleeds, and I would rather have them use it than poke me 5 times trying to get another one to bleed. The results would take a couple of weeks to come back. There has never been a question in my mind that I would develop some form of cancer. It has always been a matter of when and what kind.

Family History of Cancer

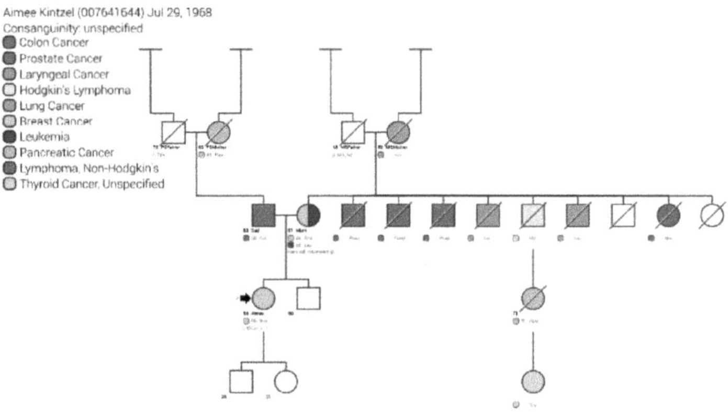

Maternal Grandmother - Lung Cancer

Mother - Breast Cancer and Hairy Cell Leukemia (twice)

3 Maternal Uncles - Prostate Cancer

1 Maternal Uncle - Laryngeal Cancer

1 Maternal Uncle - Hodgkin’s Lymphoma

1 Maternal Uncle - Lung Cancer

1 Maternal Aunt - Non-Hodgkin’s Lymphoma

1 Maternal Cousin - Pancreatic Cancer

1 Maternal Cousin - Breast Cancer (Recent enough it did not appear in my pedigree)

1 Maternal 2nd Cousin - Thyroid Cancer

Paternal Grandmother - Pancreatic Cancer

Father - Colon Cancer

Chapter 7

Aruba, Jamaica

Oooo I Wanna Take Ya.... Kokomo

The breast MRI was scheduled quickly as I have found most everything in this medical community has been. I like that. I think I mentioned I am not patient.

Somewhere along the way, I have spent time updating friends and family about what is going on. As I'm telling my 82 and 83-year-old parents about this breast MRI, my dad asks, what is special about this machine? Can you imagine? Talking about your boobs to your elderly FATHER? I explained that, basically, there would be holes cut out so my boobs would hang down and nothing would obstruct the view. I was close.

I did not want to make Jim or Betsy take more time off work, especially knowing we had many more days ahead that I would need somebody with me, so I initially planned to drive myself the hour-long drive to Kokomo, Indiana. Again, I wasn't going to learn anything at this appointment, and I wasn't going to be sedated. But, again, my support system had different ideas. I finally asked Angela if she wanted to take me. She is a local realtor, and as long as she is not showing a home or having a closing, she can pretty much make her own hours. She was happy to take m. On the way, she handed me a bag from a local jewelry store. She said to me, "I am not a good friend." I just gave her a funny look, and she went on, "I will not call and bug you, checking on you constantly, but this is to let you know I am always thinking about you." I opened the package, and inside was a beautiful necklace signifying my journey. Have I mentioned I have an amazing support system? I put the necklace on when I got home and never took it off again until immediately before my first surgery.

The procedure went off without a hitch. They took me to a room where I changed into a surgical gown and pants… huge pants. I am 5' 1" and a little overweight (ok, ok, more than a little), but WOW. Good thing they had a drawstring. After I was all changed and had my bladder empty, they took me to another anteroom where they accessed a vein (on the first stick, in the top of my hand) and started the IV fluids. The machine itself is much like any other MRI machine. However, you don't lie on a flatbed. You lie on your stomach with only a steel beam that comes between your breasts. The first couple of minutes, you think, "this is a breeze." After a few more minutes, it begins to get pretty uncomfortable. The technicians are in an adjacent room and they communicate through an intercom system the whole time. Then, when you are close to being done, they give you a warning and shoot the contrast dye through. It felt a little cold, and they said it might be uncomfortable, but I didn't have any adverse reactions. About this time (approximately twenty minutes in), my mind starts to think about my Restless Leg Syndrome. The power of suggestion made me want to move my legs, which made me even more uncomfortable. Overall, it was not bad, although they had told me if I could get through this one I could get through any MRI.

It wasn't too long before the results appeared in the MyChart app on my phone and everything appeared to be as previously suggested. The small tumor in my left breast. No lymph nodes appeared to be affected. My right breast was clear.

I then received a call from my breast surgeon's office in Anderson. Armed with the results of the MRI, she scheduled me for a lumpectomy on August 30, 2024. There would be some pre-op appointments to place markers, etc. It was a whirlwind and it was confusing. I pretty much relied on MyChart to tell me when the next appointment was scheduled.

Chapter 8

Genetics Schmenetics

While the surgeon was planning for surgery at the end of August, the results of my genetic testing came back. We tested 60 genes for possible issues. As it turned out, I have a mutation in my CHEK2 gene. This is defined as: *A Chek2 mutation is a genetic alteration in the CHEK2 gene, which plays a role in DNA damage repair and cell cycle control.* Dumbing it down: basically, this increases my risk for certain types of cancers, including breast and colon. Both of which we have established I have a predisposition to through family history. So the odds of me developing breast cancer again, even after a lumpectomy and radiation and possibly chemotherapy, were higher than the average person. I was not surprised by this. The only thing that surprised me was that out of 60 genes, only one showed a mutation. I was never really on board with that lumpectomy anyway!

I got a call from Dr. Beauty's nurse to discuss this information. The nurse explained that we could still do the lumpectomy and go that route. They almost certainly still do radiation. Possibly chemotherapy. She also explained that my follow-ups would be pretty extreme and frequent. I would have to have a breast MRI every six months, regular blood work, and some other stuff I can't remember. My mind was already thinking, "Nope. Just hack 'em off like I said in the beginning." We chatted a little more, and then she asked me what my thoughts were. Without hesitation or discussing it with anybody, I made a decision right then and there to have a total bilateral mastectomy (both breasts are removed entirely). I knew Jim would support whatever decision I made. I told the nurse it just made sense to remove all of the offending tissue! (Just hack 'em off). She was happy to hear this and said the doctor would be glad I came to that decision as well. She totally let me come to it on my own before she agreed that it would be their recommendation.

So, now the August 30 surgery was no longer on the books, and I would be sent to a plastic surgeon to talk about reconstruction after surgery. The nurse said they had a great doctor in Indianapolis that they worked with who came to Anderson once a month to work with them. She would schedule a consultation appointment with him and then get me on the books for surgery.

Chapter 9

Paging Dr Cutie

I had looked the Doctor up before we went to our appointment. This is a man very close to our daughter's age, just a couple of years older and very cute. If only he weren't married and our daughter engaged. Isn't it every mother's dream for her daughter to marry a doctor? Just kidding, Justin! I just want her to be happy!

We traveled to Indianapolis to yet another facility within the medical network on August 27, 2024. As with all the previous appointments, I was taken to the room, given a robe, and instructed to put it on "open in front." Thanks, I think I've got that by now. So I disrobe again. I shake my boobies in front of Jim again. And we wait. It's a short wait until this young man in a seersucker suit walks in, and Jim and I look at each other like, "What the fuck have we gotten ourselves into." We are country folks. We wear blue jeans and Purdue sweatshirts. We're trusting this man with the reconstruction of Jim's fun bags. Not that seersucker is bad, but seriously. Did he just come from the golf course? Maybe he did, maybe he didn't, but first impressions can be shattered. We made some small talk, mostly about the Purdue sweatshirt. Dr. Cutie, as he is now dubbed, is an IU graduate. IU has been having a phenomenal football season, and Purdue, not so much. We chatted about this at some point during most of my visits.

My plastic surgeon was very concise and to the point and said some more words we didn't really understand, but as he continued to talk, Jim and I both began to relax and believe we were right where we belonged. I asked some questions about how radiation would work if it would be before or after reconstruction. He explained to me that we very likely would not need the radiation since we would be doing the mastectomy. My guess is he could see I was a little confused. He looked at me and said, "I'm going to tell you something that goes against everything you've ever been told." He told me to relax and not try to plan ahead. He said we don't know what we are going to find at any given time and that if we try to make a solid plan, we will just be disappointed when those plans have to change. That made a lot of sense, and I have adopted it as my mantra throughout this journey. Just go with the flow.

I have had a number of people tell me about using your own fat to rebuild your breasts, and I actually did a little research. I thought this would be a great way to get rid of some extra weight. Dr. Cutie told me that was one option but that he would recommend implants instead. He said if it were his wife, he would tell her to go with implants. He said the cost was way more when using your own fat, in more ways than one. Surgery was longer when using your own tissue, recovery was longer, and it was more expensive… as well as more painful. I told him I was going to trust him, and that was that.

Somewhere during the conversation, he mentioned he would use a dead person's tissue or cadaver tissue. Wait! WHAT? As I began to gather my bottom jaw up off the floor, he explained that this tissue is stripped of any DNA and used in implant-based breast reconstruction. It is called Alloderm (or ADM-acellular dermal matrix). OK, kinda creeping me out, but again, you're the one with the diplomas; I'm going to trust you!

We talked some more about my medical history. He noted I am a former smoker and asked about that. I told him I had actually been doing a little bit of smoking recently due to stress. We talked about that, and he told me that he wanted me to stop completely. He did not lecture me about it but explained that while the media exploits the lung cancer aspect of smoking, he feels the cardiovascular repercussions are more relevant. He told us that smoking causes blood vessels to constrict, causing a significant reduction in blood flow. Reduced blood flow can cause delayed healing. I wanted this over with as quickly as possible, so I vowed not to touch another cigarette, and so far, I haven't, though it's been tempting at times.

Then, it was time to get uncomfortable. You would think I would be getting used to this by now. Maybe later! The doctor had brought his physician's assistant along with him. She was a cute young thing as well. They began measuring my breasts top to bottom and side to side, comparing one to the other. They told me that they were very symmetrical (whatever that means). Jim and I laughed about that on the way home. Maybe that would make them easier to rebuild. While I stood there getting my boobs pushed up and pulled down and moved to the left and moved to the right, Jim was sitting right there, eyes at boob level, laser-focused on what was happening. As this cute young man fondled my breasts with my husband watching, I was somewhat mortified. I looked around the room, thinking, "Where the fuck do I look?" I can't look at Jim, I can't look at the doctor, and I can't look at the physician's assistant. It does get less mortifying in time.

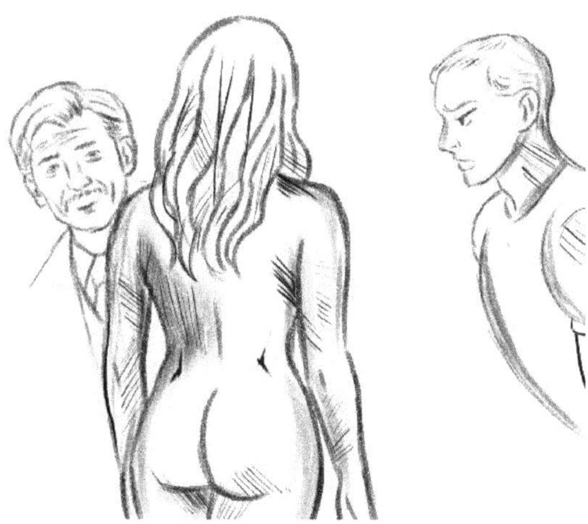

The doctor then explained that we would come for an appointment prior to surgery, and he would mark my breasts. He then said they were going to take some pictures of my breasts for reference, and as I stood there holding my gown open facing front, turning right, and then turning left, he asked who I had brought with me that day. He was referring to Jim. I forgot to mention that we jumped right into the appointment and did not make introductions. I assumed this was his way of attempting to make the situation a little less uncomfortable. I decided to be a wise guy and said, “Hell, if I know, he followed me in from the parking lot.” It took a moment, and then we all laughed.

My first appointment with the plastic surgeon was complete. It started a little bumpy, but we made it through.

On our way out of the office, I noticed a pamphlet for 3D nipple tattoos. It is a specialized procedure and not just a regular tattoo. The facility listed was in the Indianapolis area, so I decided I would try to find somebody closer that did them. Jim and I talked about it and he didn’t think it was necessary. But we were just starting this journey so maybe we would talk about it again later.

I got a call from the breast surgeon's office a few days later. Surgery was now scheduled for October 4, 2024. She didn’t come right out and say it, but the breast surgeon's nurse gave me the impression that Dr. Cutie had put it off not until the next time he was in Anderson but the time after that in order for me to get all the nicotine through my system. These people really were looking out for me.

Chapter 10

Pinterest, Google, Amazon, and the Furniture Store

I decided from the beginning that I was not going to consult with Dr. Google. That does nothing but create questions and panic. We had assembled what I was certain was an amazing team. I trusted them and believed they would tell me anything I needed to know. However, I would consult Google and Pinterest to understand how other women had handled their own journeys. I saw a lot of products recommended. Some I felt were relevant, some I did not feel I would need. I pinned information about what to take to the hospital and what to have handy at home for my recovery. I also found, on Pinterest, a wonderful group that provides heart-shaped pillows at no cost to the patient. You just email them your story, and the next thing you know you are receiving a package in the mail. They do ask for donations to help with postage/shipping costs, and as it turned out, the founder's daughter has written a book she will try to sell you without pressure, but hey…free pillows, and I am still using them.

I got on Amazon and started buying. I started with zip-front shirts with pockets on the inside for drain tubes. These came highly recommended but were expensive. I shopped around, and they ranged from $19.99 up to the $40's. I bought them as inexpensively as I could since I would be wearing them for only a brief period of time. I also bought lounge pants to match. Because… you have to match! I am so glad I purchased those tops. Having the pockets for drain tubes was such a convenience. I had an apron with pockets for when I did not have pockets in my shirts. It did the trick but was in the way. I am still using the lounge pants, so win-win. I purchased a "mastectomy pillow," which was pretty much a 3 section pillow.

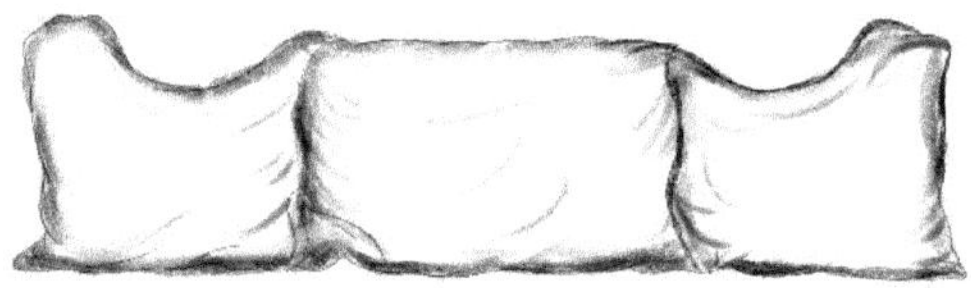

The front had pockets for incidentals, like a book, your cell phone, or a snack, so you could keep them handy. Each side had a cutout area for the arms. It had straps, and it fastened on. This would become my best friend. I ordered bath wipes because I would not be allowed to shower for a day or two. I bought books to read and puzzle books as well as snacks. This was all suggested in a what-to bring-to-the-hospital pin. Hindsight is 20/20. I did not need books, reading or otherwise. Maybe if my stay had been longer and I needed to entertain myself throughout the day I might have used more of this stuff. I did not use the bath wipes. But they are coming in handy with the messy grandson. I really didn't care whether or not I stunk. And I didn't touch the snacks until I was home. I was provided breakfast in the hospital the morning after my surgery, and then we were headed home shortly after that. I had received a bag full of goodies from a very generous group that provides them to the hospital to give to mastectomy patients. I also received two camisoles through my surgeon's office that had velcro closures in the front and pockets so I could stash my drain tubes while in pajamas. My advice? Do your research. Understand what you will want/need and plan appropriately. Don't be afraid to ask what is provided by your surgeon's office or the hospital. I am glad I was over-prepared and not underprepared, but I took way more stuff than I needed, and somebody just had to drag it all home.

Another thing I learned through my Pinterest investigation was that I would not be able to sleep flat. I knew I wouldn't be sleeping on my side or stomach like I am accustomed to, but this was fairly unexpected. People recommended renting a recliner if you did not already have one. I had one that was very comfortable and great for sleeping. But the reclining lever was on the side. I think I've mentioned that I am vertically challenged, and I could not imagine having to reach over the side to pull that lever to recline or un-recline. So off to the furniture store we went. We found a double recliner with a console in the middle. It is electronic, and the control is in the console of each arm. We had been contemplating getting one for a while. Perfect. No reaching. We tested it in the furniture store, but apparently, we didn't do as much sitting or reclining as we should have. Once we had it in our home, we learned it was not the most comfortable piece of furniture we had ever had. The backrest is a bit too forward and is no fun on the neck, and it doesn't recline as far as we would like. The footrest comes up first then the back reclines. So, if we wanted to adjust it for our neck, we had to have our feet up. But this was going to be my home for a while, so we made the best of it and enjoyed not having to reach over to recline. Don't feel like you have to go get new furniture. It worked out for us as we needed something new anyway. Otherwise, I would have made do with what we had. Again, do your own research. Don't stress about needing to buy a bunch of stuff. This was my way of keeping my mind occupied so that I did not overthink and worry.

And just because I could, I bought a few more front-opening tops for after surgery. I was stylin' and ready.

Chapter 11
The Things You Don't Think About

There are a lot of things you don't even think about. We like to see our favorite band, Tesla, whenever they are playing anywhere close. We especially enjoy visiting different venues. Jim has seen them in concert a dozen or more times, and I am at least half that many. We like to say that Chad has been to one of their concerts because we went to one when I was pregnant with him.

We were scheduled to go to a new venue to see them on September 25, 2024. We had great seats. Because I always get on early and purchase the best seats we can afford. If I can't have good seats, why bother? I am short, and once everybody stands up, I can't see. So the third row it was.

We decided the week of the concert that we did not want to risk me picking up a germ and getting sick so close to surgery. I didn't want anything to delay it. So we decided not to attend. It was a hard decision to make, but in the grand scheme of things, we have seen them… and will again, and my health was not worth it. We tried to sell the tickets, but it was short notice, and the concert was on Wednesday night. We couldn't even give them away. Even though it bummed us out, I am certain it was the right decision. I saw a lot of Facebook posts about it afterward and heard it was a kick-ass show, as always!

We don't go out much anyway, except for our concerts, but we found ourselves avoiding going out and spending time with people more and more in the days leading up to surgery. I even started ordering my groceries to be delivered right to my front door. I just didn't want to take the chance of having to postpone surgery. I wanted that shit out of my body!

Another thing to be considered is that I cut my dad's hair every few months. He has not been to a barber since COVID-19 hit. He refused to wear a mask. So he went for 6 months without a haircut until they returned from Florida that year. So began Aimee's Barber Shop. I made sure I got over to their house and got his hair cut right before surgery because we didn't know how long it would be until I would be able to do it again. He then would not let me do it again until I was completely released from restrictions after my reconstruction surgery. October to January without a haircut can make a man pretty shaggy. Eyebrown and ear hair on a man his age can get pretty unruly.

How would Bennett react? Mimi likes to get on the floor and roughhouse with him. He was only 4 years old. How could he understand that Mimi could no longer do this? I roughhoused with him as much as I could stand leading up to my surgery.

Jim has a barnyard full of animals. I would not be spending any time with him out there. I would not be available to help him in a hurry-up situation. It was a good thing Chad was living with us at the time because he would be called on more than once to help his dad.

I wouldn't be able to cook or clean. The cooking was taken care of by our amazing support system. But how was Jim going to be able to work a full-time job, handle his chores, take care of me, AND keep up with the laundry and dishes? I tried to get as much done ahead as I could, but these things tend to keep needing to be done. He did it.

I wouldn't be going on any adventures for a while. This meant no trips to the casino, no spur-of-the-moment trips to the craft stores or my favorite restaurants. I tried to get some lunches in with friends prior, and stocked up on some craft supplies. Little did I know I would not be using them for a while.

I would not be driving. Remember that independence I talked about? Out the door! I would not be able to jump in the car and run to the grocery store or pharmacy.

I think I mentioned Jim and I are an amorous couple. Prior to this, we had never gone more than two weeks without being intimate. That included after the birth of each of our children and him spending two weeks in the hospital for a ruptured appendix (yes, the day I brought him home).

I love me a nice hot soaking bubble bath. I did not realize it, but I would not be able to do that for a long time. Longer than just my initial recovery.

The list could go on. Just keep in mind that anything that required lifting my arms and/or repetitive movement was out of the question, as was lifting any amount of weight.

The biggest thing I was not prepared for was the total exhaustion. I knew I would be wiped out while I was taking pain medications during my initial recovery. But going back to work was way more taxing than I expected it would be. By the afternoon of my first day, I was hurting. Not bad, just enough to let me know I had just been through major surgery 3 weeks prior, and I was so tired I could barely keep my eyes open. My amazing work family could see that I was struggling and urged me to go home. I made it home that afternoon and slept. This exhaustion would continue far longer than I would have expected. Even after I was able and feeling better, I did not go on any of my spur-of-the-moment excursions because I did not want to hold anybody else up or make them have to come home early. We didn't go out for dinners, and definitely no parties. I did go to the big CASA fundraiser exactly 4 weeks after my mastectomy. While it was a fun night, and all I had to do was relax and have fun, it wore me out. It is a big event with a big crowd. I was more than ready to go home at the end of the night. I would get tired so easily and so early. It got to the point I felt like people were going to think I was just using it as an excuse. I wasn't, and nobody ever accused me of it… that I know of, but when you are accustomed to being the Energizer Bunny and all of a sudden your batteries don't last, it can throw you for a loop. At times, I still find myself more tired than I feel like I should be, but I just remind myself that I need to slow down. Anything that needs to be done can wait until I take a brief siesta.

My house still isn't where I would like it to be as far as clutter and cleanliness, but I find a little more energy each day and it will get there.

Chapter 12

The Countdown Begins

On the Tuesday night before my surgery on Friday, my phone rang at approximately 8:00 p.m., knowing Dr. Beauty, the breast surgeon, wanted to chat with me prior to surgery. I answered the call even though I did not recognize the number. She explained how everything would go. She said it would take 3-4 hours. She would go in and do her part, and when she was finished with one side, Dr. Cutie would be called in to start putting me back together on that side while she finished up on the other. She would then go out and talk to my family, and then he would when he was done. She told me I would spend one night in the hospital, barring complications. I would likely have drain tubes, but she couldn't tell me how many or how long I would have those. She explained that she would take some lymph nodes along with the breast tissue. She told me that the tumor would then be sent for testing. This would determine whether or not there would be a need for chemotherapy later. She was very thorough. She answered all of my questions. She asked me if I had any more questions and I told her I did not. She then said she just had one more thing to say. She told me that they would take care of me and that I did not need to worry about anything. To that, I responded that I was not at all worried, that we felt pretty certain that we were in good hands, and that my husband, who would rather see a veterinarian than a doctor, even liked the team we had assembled. She laughed and said I had made her night and that she would see me on Friday. I am a nervous person by nature. I worry about everything and overthink anything that can be overthought. This! This life-changing surgery did not make me worry or fret! I felt certain from the beginning I was going to be alright. Once we assembled our team, I had no doubts.

Two days prior to my surgery, we traveled to Indianapolis for my "mapping." The doctor used a purple marker to draw circles around my boobs and lines through them. For us, it looked like he was just scribbling, but I am sure it was telling Dr. Beauty where to cut (how to take me apart) and him how to put me back together. He then sent us home with two of those little markers in case his coloring faded. I had instructions to wash my entire torso with a special antibacterial, antiseptic soap for the two days prior to and on the morning of surgery. So, yes, the lines faded. It was difficult for me to draw over the lines while looking in the mirror, and Jim's hands shook, so we made quite the pair with this task. We were able to keep the lines visible enough though. Whew!

Chapter 13
Family, Friends, and Work Family

Once we had a plan, we updated work and family with the date for my first surgery. On another visit with my parents, we talked about the surgery and what I would be expecting. Remember the conversation with my dad about the breast MRI machine? That was only half as mortifying as the conversation we had during this visit. So, I don't recall telling my mom that I may lose my nipples, but apparently, she has ascertained this information from somewhere. Because my dad blurted out, "Your mom says you're not going to have any nipples." As calmly as I could, I explained that this was a possibility. I really wished I could crawl under the table. Seriously though. He was concerned and wanted to know whatever he could. I love my parents dearly! But some conversations are just awkward.

I also took some time to tell a group of our longtime friends. We are four couples, and some of us have been friends for over 40 years. Our children all grew up together. They are family. We don't get together as often as we would like, but when we do, we laugh… a lot, often about the same stupid stories from back in the day. I wanted them to know. I didn't want to spring it on them if they wanted to get together one night. That was all I told. There are a lot more people I could have and perhaps should have told, but I was done talking about it and just wanted to be looking at the whole thing in the rearview mirror. I learned later that Jim had told pretty much everyone he had encountered since day one. That's fine. He needed to talk about it. I didn't. We all respond differently. There is no right or wrong to how you deal with something like this. Just do your best to deal with it as it comes. Make no apologies to anybody for how you handle it. This is your journey!

My work family is amazing. I started a new job in February, so I had been with them for only 6 months at the time of my diagnosis. While it was really bothering me to be off work so much, everyone was always encouraging and positive. When this journey first started, I asked my immediate supervisor not to say anything to anybody until I knew what was going on. Through the ultrasound and biopsy, she kept it just between us. Even after my diagnosis, we kept it between us until after my first visit with the oncologist and the whirlwind of appointments started. I gave her permission to share at that point. I cannot begin to explain the outpouring of love I received from this group. Hugs, encouragement, prayers, and even some tears. My coworkers regularly asked about any updates and how I was feeling. As I shared each update, we laughed together about the many things I found humorous.

The day before surgery came, and I walked into work to a party just for me. There was food and balloons and a T-shirt and pink hat for me. I went and changed into my black and pink warrior t-shirt and wore my sparkly pink hat all day long. Everyone was wearing pink in some form. More hugs, more prayers, and more encouragement. They had also planned a meal train for us. We would not go hungry for a while.

My former employer works in the same building, and she brought me a big bag of goodies, including snacks, books, and a blanket that I slept with every day and night through my recovery.

I really felt the love when I walked out of work that day.

I can honestly say that these are my people! Coworkers and friends, all of whom have become FAMILY.

Chapter 14
Surgery #1

Surgery day came, and we traveled to Anderson. GPS took us in a slightly different direction, but we learned that this was because the hospital entrance was on the other side of the building from the surgeon's office. Again, it was easy to get to and easy to get into. We didn't argue about where to enter this time. It was pretty obvious. We got checked in, and Jim was given information about how he could follow how the surgery was going on the airport arrivals and departures board. I was taken back to get prepped. An IV line was started. I did warn them I would be their challenge for the day, but they were champs and got me stuck on the first try. I was put into the bed. Jim was brought back, and we texted everyone back home to let them know how things were going.

Nuclear medicine came in to give me an injection that would show the surgeon which lymph nodes my breast drained into and, thus, which ones to remove. The nurse/technician walked in with literally a lead pipe in her hand. There was a syringe in it filled with whatever it was they shot into me. She would inject this, and then we would wait 30 minutes or so then take x-rays. The needle going in was fine, but that shit they shot into me hurt! I winced and told the technician that I guessed I wasn't as much of a badass as I thought I was. She said that even the toughest-looking gals struggled with this. I was sure glad that was over. When it was time to go for the x-ray, they came in with a funky wheelchair that was supposed to be easier to get into than a conventional one. I felt that it was not. I am a clutz, though. Maybe that had something to do with it. I am certain the x-ray tech thought she was in a NASCAR race because I'm pretty sure I was close to falling out through a couple of corners. We made it safely, and I got up on the table, and we got the pictures. Then, back through the racetrack, we went back to my bed.

At one point, the anesthesiologist came in to explain what he would be doing. Another young, cute fella. Maybe I just think everybody's cute at this point. He was a character. He told me he had looked up what he needed to do on YouTube that morning and felt pretty confident that he could handle it. I laughed and tried to make a joke that would make it clear I was not offended and understood he was joking. Nothing would come to mind. Oh well! I guess I'm not as funny as I think I am.

We were told that my surgeons were running a little behind but that they were there and ready to do their things when they were done with the surgery ahead of me. We waited. Fortunately, there was a bathroom right next door, and I used it often. I call it my old lady/mom bladder. Add nerves, and I had to pee a lot. On my final trip to empty the bladder, I had a new tech helping me. Dr. Cutie was just coming in to tell me that they were done and getting ready for me. We got into the bathroom, and the tech, who was not only new to me but new to the hospital, asked me, "WHO WAS THAT?" Since he only came to this hospital once a month, she had not yet met him. I laughed and told her he was just the guy who was gonna rebuild my boobs.

Finally, they came to take me back. Jim stood up, kissed me, and we said our "I Love You's" and started to cry. I admonished him and told him to stop it, and everyone laughed at us. He was far more nervous than I was. After that nuclear medicine injection, I wasn't really afraid of anything. I was just going to go take a nice nap.

In the operating room, I got onto the operating table and spread my arms to my sides. The anesthesiologist at my head started his YouTube routine again, and I drifted off to sleep with the assistants in the room giggling and telling me he was very good and not to worry. I wasn't worried.

About 20 minutes later (not really) I woke up. I don't remember much about recovery. But I know that when I got to my suite, Erin was with Jim. She had made the trip down after working all day. Surgery had actually taken close to six hours. I had four drain tubes. Margins were good (more words! Basically, she got enough tissue around the tumor itself. We would most likely not need the radiation.) She took out three lymph nodes. I had tissue expanders where my breasts had been.

Anybody who has ever been in a hospital knows I did not sleep much that night, nor did Erin, who was trying to sleep on the sofa in my room. I said I had a suite. There was even a kitchenette.

Dr. Beauty, the breast surgeon, had told me when we were prepping for surgery that she had a prior engagement the next day and would send someone to check on me in the morning. She was to be in Indianapolis to participate in a Breast Cancer benefit fashion show by 7:00 a.m. I woke up around 5:00 a.m. or so to this beautiful young lady dressed to the nines standing over me. After performing two major surgeries and not getting out of the hospital until after 9:00 p.m. the day before, she had gotten up extra early to check on me. She said she just couldn't begin her day without checking on me herself. She was pleased with what she saw and said she would see me in a week or so.

Before I could leave, we had to learn how to empty my drain tubes and how to keep track of the output. I was afraid this would gross me out, so I made them wait for my farmer husband to get back. He said he could handle anything with his farm animals, but he didn't think he would be able to do this with me. Erin watched, too, just in case she needed to help. Everything must have been hunky dory because that was the only thing we needed to do before I could come home.

I got dressed in one of my zip-front shirts and ever so carefully tucked my drains into the pockets inside. Armed with my Amazon purchases and all the other goodies I had received, we headed home.

Chapter 15
Home

With my new best friend attached to the front of me, we strapped me into the car and headed home. I think I read a little on the way home, but it was an otherwise uneventful drive. As soon as we got home, I changed into pajamas and headed for the couch. Jim was so attentive, brought me my medications on schedule, and left me to sleep unless I asked him for something. My mom wanted to help. She came bearing one of my all-time favorite meals that afternoon: Martha Leek's chicken pie (not to be confused with anybody's chicken pot pie), mashed potatoes, and gravy. She wanted so badly to help with some chores but had to keep asking me questions, and I had to keep getting up. I finally told her that her just being there and visiting would be enough. After a bit, she left, and I slept. I developed a schedule where I took my meds and slept for a couple of hours at a time.

Jim stayed home with me for the first week and a half. I couldn't have asked for better care. When you get married, you agree to love each other through sickness and health. He definitely lived up to that vow. He would empty my drains in the morning, bring my medications on schedule, and then leave me alone unless I needed something. We have a small farm, and he would go out and spend time with his cattle but checked on me often. He got to meet many of my new work family members when they would bring food. Then, we would empty the drains again before bed at night.

I was very surprised that I did not have a lot of pain. Mostly discomfort. Jim was amazed by this as well and would tell many people how surprised he was that I didn't have more issues. Perhaps that was the good medications they gave me and keeping on schedule before they could wear off. But seriously. I felt like this had pretty much been a breeze. Of course, I slept through the 6 hours of surgery while my family worried. This entire ordeal has been way worse for them than I feel like it has been for me.

I was given permission to shower 48 hours post-surgery. I desperately wanted to, but Jim was not ready. He knew he would need to help me, and he was terrified of hurting me. I finally talked him into letting me a day or two later. I took one of the good pills, and off we went. We hadn't really had my breasts uncovered completely up to this point. He had not seen my incision lines, and his reaction was a little unnerving. I hadn't looked at them at all at this point and still didn't. I just wasn't ready. I got into the shower while Jim waited. Apparently, my medication kicked in while I was in the shower, and I became "chatty." Jim called it mouthy. He told me it was time to get out because he was afraid I was going to fall.

Jim would not let me wash my hair and wouldn't do it for me because he didn't want to hurt me during that first shower, so my hair went unwashed. I commented in our work family text group that I really wanted to wash my hair. One of my amazing co-workers brought me a waterless hair cleaner. It looked like a shower cap, and you put it on your head and massage it. It felt so good. I wasn't yet allowed to raise my arms, so my amazing sidekick had to do all of this. Then we took it off, and he combed my hair. I felt incredible. My hair looked and smelled so much better. However, it wasn't long before it wore off, and I really needed to take another shower and wash it with shampoo and water.

Friends and family came and went and brought food or whatever they thought we might need. I binge-watched Dexter and developed an online shopping problem. I would need to get back to work soon, to support it. Jim did his best to keep up with housework, but between working his full-time (and then some) job, his animals, and taking care of me, he was pretty busy. The clutter began to drive me crazy.

I was given a list of restrictions. I could not lift my arms up at all, and I could not lift any weight. I could not push or pull anything. I was not allowed to do any repetitive movements. I was determined to heal fast and well, so I did NOTHING but sleep, eat, and watch television (and shop online). One of my favorite ways to pass the time is to crochet or craft in general. I thought I might do some of that while I was home, but with no repetitive movements, that was out of the question.

Chad came in with his little boy, Bennett (the four-year-old), for his first visit after my surgery. They stopped at the door, and I heard them whispering. Bennett was so gentle with me, and it killed me not being able to rough house with him. I would usually get on the floor and play with him whenever he was around, whether it be Lego's, magnet tiles, or coloring. Now, I could not get up and down and could not play with him. He would not hug me straight on or climb into my lap. And he always, always asked if I was "still hurt." Bennett would tell anybody who came over while he was there that Mimi was hurt and that they had to be quiet and gentle when they came in. Oh, my protective boys.

Chapter 16
First Post-OP

At about one and a half weeks, both surgeon's offices had scheduled post-operative visits on different days. The breast surgeon's nurse was awesome and was able to change the appointment there to the same day as the plastic surgeon. So we traveled to Anderson.

The nurse prepared me for drain tube removal, but the surgeon decided to let the plastic surgeon's office do that. She told us everything looked great and that she did not need to see me again. She was very happy with my healing. She told me that even though they did not need to see me, I should feel free to call them anytime with any concerns. She explained that I would no longer get mammograms but that I would have a manual breast exam. She said if at any time something is found and I want her to check it out, I could reach out to them. I could not have asked for a better breast surgeon for this part of my journey. The receptionist handed me a small gift bag on my way out, and my time in Anderson was complete.

After that appointment, we drove further south to Indianapolis to see the plastic surgeon for my first post-op appointment there. The nurse took us into the room. We talked about drain tubes and where we were with the output. One on each side was putting out little enough that they could be removed. She prepared with bandages and started pulling. Boy, I did not realize how far those tubes went. I was sure I could feel them coming out of my brain. It was not painful, but I could feel them tugging. Just a weird feeling. She bandaged me up and told me to check them and put antibiotic ointment and a new bandage on each of the next couple of days or until they looked like they were closed.

Shortly after that, the physician's assistant and a medical student came in and started setting things up so that my tissue expanders could be filled. As it turns out, when they put tissue expanders in, they are filled with air. They need to suck this air out and fill them with saline. The saline bag was hung, and a syringe was set out. They asked if either of us was squeamish, and I explained that while I could be, he was a farm boy and could handle most anything. She explained that they had a patient who had brought her older mother with her. She had not been prepared for the result after deflation. We were prepared. I was deflated. I didn't think it was gross or anything like that, but wow did it look different when I looked down. Crazy sensation.

The doctor came in and explained what was going to happen. He stated that there was a port, very much like a chemo port, in each breast that was "self-healing.". I told him that I had wondered how he was going to poke a hole in them and fill them with saline and not expect them to leak. I guessed now I knew.

Using the same syringe that was used to suck the air out, they began pushing saline into my tissue expanders. From what I understand, this is often done in steps, but we were going for a Hail Mary and doing it all in one visit. Since we were going big (because fat Aimee had big ones), there was a lot of saline pushing. Their hands were getting tired. By the time they finished with one side, the doctor had decided to use a "four-pronger." Ok, seriously. You've already stuck a big needle into my boob, and now you're coming at me with a serving fork. I asked what the reason was, and everybody but me said so we could fill it 4 times faster. OK, dude, next time, let me know, and I'll bring my own fork. If you're going to use a four-pronger every time, I'm glad we did it all in one shot.

As with most of my appointments here, we talked about college football and music, and Jim, thinking it was somewhat disturbing, told him about my addiction to Dexter. He thought that was cool and wondered where I was in the series. We discussed our favorite characters, and he told me to watch and see if I could figure out when the lead actors, who had gotten married a couple of seasons in, got divorced.

I had hoped to go back to work after two weeks because some of the things I was reading said I might be able to. I felt great, had little to no pain, and only took the good medication when I wanted to sleep. I had also read, however, that I had to be drain tube-free before I would be allowed to drive. So, I began to diligently watch the output from these drains. Finally, on Friday, October 25, exactly 3 weeks after my surgery, I felt like the output was low enough that I could get the last two removed. I called Angela and asked her if she wanted to take a road trip to Indianapolis. I called to let them know I was ready to get them removed and made sure somebody would be able to see me, and off we went. A different nurse and a different way of doing things. She told me to take a deep breath and just pulled it out on my exhale. While the first two, as I said, did not hurt, they felt funny, and these were far less uncomfortable. Yay, me, no more drain tubes. Truth be told, I did not once pull them or make them hurt in any way, but they were such a pain. They had to be kept secured, either in my pockets or pinned to a lanyard when I showered. Being careful was key, but between that and having to empty them twice a day, I often told people they were the bane of my existence.

To celebrate, we stopped and ate at the Cheesecake Factory for lunch.

I returned to work on Monday, October 28, with my restrictions intact. I could not lift more than 5 pounds, and I could not push or pull anything. This was a hard task for me. I am not used to asking for help, so I would lift something up off the floor, and even if it was not heavy, I would catch Hell. This was especially difficult given that we were in the middle of an office remodel, and I had to move workstations twice during this time. But we muddled through.

Chapter 17
Louise and Roxanne

It was during the trip to get my drain tubes out that Angela began to tell me that she felt like Lefty Louise was smaller than Roxanne. I told her it was no big deal; these were still just my tissue expanders, and I wasn't worried about them being even. She persisted every time we saw each other after that. I began to look closer and discovered that Lefty was not necessarily smaller but had shifted. I began holding my arm under my left breast to "keep her in place." I'm sure I looked like I had an injured arm. Suppose that's what people thought, oh well. At least I didn't have to explain it. I would often joke about my wandering boob. I decided I would address this at my next appointment.

In mid-November, I had another post-operative appointment. I was sitting there in my robe (open in front), and the doctor came in. He asked how things were going. I told him, "I have questions." He told me, "ok, shoot." I opened the left side of my robe and asked him, "What the hell is going on with this one?" He said, "Let me see the other one for comparison." I opened the other side, and he made a noise that assured me this was not normal. But HE assured me that he had seen it before and he was not worried. He said a stitch inside had most likely come loose. They would fix it when they did my implant placement surgery. "Next question…Why does it hurt when I reach the littlest bit with my right arm?" "There is probably a stitch pulling." Next question, "Can I sleep in my bed?" He replied that he was surprised I wasn't already, and my last question was, could I take a bath? He told me no to that one because there was a very small spot that wasn't completely healed. He advised me to slather it with Vaseline and put a bandage over it until it looked like it was completely healed. Not to worry! I would do whatever I needed to. I wanted that bubble bath.

We talked about when we might schedule the next surgery. He said he would prefer to wait and check that spot for healing one more time. He told me I could probably twist his arm if I really wanted to, and I told him he was the one with the degrees and medical license. I would trust him. So, we would make at least one more trip to Indianapolis before surgery was scheduled. On December 3, we made our final trip, prior to reconstruction, to Indianapolis. The spot had healed, and he would have his scheduler call. A few days passed, and I had not heard from her, so I tried calling. I got a voicemail message that stated it could take up to 14 days to get the surgery scheduled. I had medication that I could not take for 2 weeks prior to surgery, so I waited only a few more days and called again. I apologized, stating that I understood she was probably swamped with people trying to get on the schedule before the end of the year but that I needed to know whether or not I could take my medication. She understood and got me scheduled for December 26.

In the meantime, Louise continued to wander, but it was just more fodder for my sense of humor.

Chapter 18

I Just Want to Feel Like Myself Again

Throughout this journey, I have not shed any tears for myself. I do not want to feel sorry for myself, and I do not want anybody else to feel sorry for me. But it seemed like all the TV shows on regular TV were having breast cancer storylines. 9-1-1 Lonestar had me sobbing one night. I commented that I don't cry for myself, but a made-up story has me sobbing, and somebody, I'm not sure who told me that was because I am traumatized. Maybe that's right, maybe not, but I found it so odd.

Eventually, I felt that I needed a "poor me" day. The tissue expanders were incredibly uncomfortable, and with Louise continuing to wander, I was frustrated. I just wanted this to be over. I just wanted to feel like myself. Those tissue expanders are made of something very strong, and the only way I could explain what they feel like inside your chest is by using one of those heavy plastic reusable shopping bags. Jim was still afraid to touch me. He wasn't afraid of popping one of those expanders, but knowing how uncomfortable they were, he was afraid he was going to hurt me. I was down but still not crying. This is significant because I am a Cryer. I cry at commercials.

I expressed my frustration to Jim, who just sort of blew it off. I became more frustrated, and I finally lost it on him. I told him,

"You have babied me throughout his entire shit show, and now that I actually want you to, you don't care!" He laughed and just said, "It'll be alright." It was nothing special, nothing lovey-dovey. Nothing like the way he has treated me since the diagnosis. And that was exactly what I needed. I snapped out of it and started laughing at myself. I was still uncomfortable and I still wanted them out, but I was no longer feeling sorry for myself.

I knew of a few people close to my own age who have somewhat recently had their own battles with breast cancer. I reached out to ask them what their journeys had consisted of. The ones who had traveled the same path told me that it was normal to feel the way I did and that the expanders were the worst. They assured me that it would get better.

I felt better, and my humor returned.

Chapter 19

Follow-up treatments

So, I stated that Dr. Beauty had told me she got everything. Good margins, etc. This meant I would not need to have radiation. What we were still not sure about was chemotherapy. The tumor had been sent off for genetic testing of its own to get an "onco-type" score.

We traveled to Fort Wayne on October 21 to meet with the oncologist. She explained that if the onco-type score was 25 or higher, she would recommend that I received Chemotherapy for a specified amount of time. She told me the number of treatments and how long it would be, but I don't remember that information now.

The report dated the very next day, October 22, came back with an onco-type score of 13. NO CHEMOTHERAPY. This was such exciting news. I would not have to go through that nightmare.

I would have to continue seeing the oncologist indefinitely due to the hormone blockers I would be taking eventually. The side effects it could cause must be monitored closely.

Chapter 20
Not your typical Christmas

I had decided I would not put up a tree. I wasn't really feeling like I should, and I am the only one who really cares anyway, right? Wrong! Bennett was devastated by this thought. So I went and bought a small tree and put it in our bay window. Bennett and I do a lot of crafts together, so we made easy decorations, and he and his dad put them on. Later, I decided the clutter was making me crazy and cleaned it up one day while I binge-watched "Cobra Kai." With the space clutter-free, I decided I would put my farm-themed skinny tree up. This made Bennett quite happy when I let him help me put the decorations on. Fear not! I sat on the floor to do the declutter, and I lifted only light things, and I worked in hitches so that I did not overdo it.

Since Bennett travels between his mom's and his dad's homes, we schedule events around when he will be with us, Erin's work schedule, and Justin's family time. Bennett was going to be with us Monday night to wake up on Christmas Eve, but Erin worked on Tuesday, so we decided to have our family Christmas on Monday night, the 23rd. We had a great Christmas and a wonderful time together. Knowing that I would be sitting home on Christmas day without my family coming to celebrate, I decided to take the tree down on Christmas Eve. Bennett was in his room playing with his dad while I did that and he was not pleased when he came out. Kids apparently love their Christmas trees.

I had made a reservation in a hotel close to the hospital for Christmas night. My surgery was scheduled for early the next day, and I would need to be there by 6:45 a.m. We did not want to make the two-hour drive at that time, so we decided to travel down to Indianapolis that night. We were driving along following the GPS and saw our hotel with a construction dumpster and very few cars in the lot. We started to panic that they were closed for construction. I probably should have told you that on the night of my first surgery, I had made a reservation for Jim at a nearby hotel, but when he got there, it was not open. It was a brand-new hotel that would not open until the following Monday. I made an online reservation and received a confirmation number. We were going to be very peeved if this one wasn't open. It was. There was a lot of construction, but we were put into a newly renovated room. It was beautiful and cozy, but it had a futuristic remote for the TV that we could not operate. Minor inconveniences in the grand scheme of things.

Chapter 21

Surgery #2

It was an early morning, but we only had a 5-minute drive from the hotel. We got to the surgery center, and got all checked in. I barely sat down before a nurse called my name. She took me back for my surgery prep. She talked about the nerve block procedure that I would have and asked if I had had it prior to my first surgery. I told her I had not (I was wrong). She also told me that at this hospital, they swab your neck and feet with an antiseptic. The solution is cold and sticky, and she had a funny name for it, but I don't recall that now. She was going to start my IV. Again, I explained that I was a hard draw and that I would be her challenge for the day. They always thank me when I say that. She didn't have any trouble at all. I guess knowing is half the battle.

There was a young child I could hear crying from another room. He was very distraught and unhappy. I felt for this poor child. However, when I left my room briefly and walked directly into him while his mom was carrying him around, trying to console him, I lost it. I walked back into my room and started sobbing. He's just a little boy. He doesn't understand. I learned later he was getting tubes in his ears, which I know is generally a pretty standard and easy procedure, but like I said, he did not understand. This is a particularly interesting part of my story because I still have not cried for myself throughout this journey.

They took me back for the nerve block, which was done in a recovery room and was another somewhat painful experience. My surgeon, Dr. Cutie, came in to go over everything after I returned and told me I had, in fact, had a nerve block during the first surgery, but they did it after I was under anesthesia, so I didn't feel it. Cool! Why didn't they do that here? He said he didn't know why they did it prior to surgery at this location. We talked about Christmas and black tie events and just a lot of small talk to make us more comfortable, and then they whisked me away in the middle of his story about Valentine's Day. He told Jim he would finish it later. He never got the chance to finish.

While I was in recovery, Dr. Cutie explained to Jim that the reason Louise had wandered was because my body cannibalized the cadaver tissue (The Alloderm I thought was creepy earlier). OK, I made that up. He didn't say cannibalized, but doesn't that sound like a good story? What he actually said was that my body absorbed it faster than normal, so there was nothing there to hold the tissue expander in place. He put extra in with the implant placement. Surgery, again, went off without a hitch. I now had my new boobs. Merry Christmas to me!

Erin and I dubbed my new breasts my Christmas Knockers. She wanted to call them my Christmas titties, but I felt with no nipples, this was a bit off course. You know, because we are perfectly sane people! When my mother-in-law had her breasts removed, she did not have reconstruction. I'm not sure if it was her age or the fact that she had been on the smallish side, to begin with. They never even mentioned reconstruction to her. But she did get a padded mastectomy bra that she wears for "special occasions." We call it her Church Boobs.

I had been for two post-op visits at the plastic surgeon's office. I was seen by the physician's assistant on both occasions. There was one spot on the first visit that she wanted me to watch closely, and therefore, she told me I could not soak in the bathtub because of it. But overall, she thought everything was going well. During the second visit, she felt everything looked great. She said you couldn't even tell where Dr. Cutie had gone in through the first incision. Jim commented after we left that she really seemed to like my boobs. I think she was just proud of the work they did.

At my appointment on February 4, 2025, I was told that all restrictions were lifted. I was so excited I could now roughhouse with Bennett and have a bath. Those were my two most anticipated things. That was a Tuesday, so Bennett would come for his visit with his dad that night. I took him aside and asked him, "Guess what?" He could not guess what my news was, so I picked him up and told him, “Mimi can pick you up now.” He was so excited. He is so fun and funny. Anytime somebody he hasn’t told comes around, He will have me pick him up and tell them, “Guess what? Mimi can pick me up again.”

Chapter 22
Getting Back to Normal

I came home after my implant placement surgery, ready to hang out on the couch again. There was no overnight stay for this surgery. As soon as I was cleared from recovery, we headed home. Still a little groggy, I slept most of the way home. I changed into my pajamas and strapped my trusted best friend to my chest, got under my blanket, and planned to sleep the day away. I did sleep some, but there seemed to be more pain with this surgery than there had been with the first one. They used the same incisions, but I think I had some muscles waking up that were affected by this one. It still was not excruciating but bad enough to be annoying. It could have been the lesser-strength pain medications, too. They were still good, but not at the Opioid addiction level good. It was a little frustrating that this two-hour surgery recovery was going harder than the six-hour surgery. I was feeling a little sorry for myself again.

My boobs felt a little more normal than they had with the tissue expanders, but they felt very heavy. They are not quite as perky as I had thought (hoped) they would. I sleep on my side most of the time, and I find that the breast on the side that is down flattens and becomes horizontal with the bed. This was a little unnerving the first time I noticed, but I am getting used to that. They still do the things older women's boobs do. They lie down when I do, and they still need a little lift up off my belly. While I don't need the underwire bra anymore, I do feel like they look much better when I have a bra on. Visually, a bra is not required. Bras, bras, bras. What a pain in the ass these things are. Like I said, I don't really need one, but it's just more comfortable with one. I have found some really comfortable bras, but they don't accentuate my girls. I figured I had to go through this, and I might as well show them off. We'll find the right bra eventually.

I did lose my nipples. But my incision scars come to a point in the middle of each breast, and it looks like I have nipples. Jim likes to point this out. He comments on these "nipples" at times, and I have told him that they are not my nipples. My nipples are in a landfill somewhere. Ok, maybe it's not just some landfill somewhere, but wherever human tissue is disposed of.

Jim is no longer afraid of hurting me, and his radar and cheese-wrapper doggy sense are back. If I comment on this being different or that not being the same, he will look at me and say, "But there is no cancer." But there is no cancer. A mantra we recite often.

Sometime in early December, I got a call from a very dear longtime friend, who was extremely apologetic. She felt like she had failed me because she had not come around during my recovery or done anything to help us out.

I laughed and told her we were all busy and had lives that demanded our attention. I was not offended, nor did I feel she had neglected or failed me. She was adamant that she had been a bad friend and wanted to make up for it. She made me promise to let her know when my next surgery would be so that she could come, bring food, and do any house chores I wanted her to. I agreed to let her know as soon as I knew. I told her immediately upon scheduling my surgery. She said she would be there for the day.

She came the day of my surgery, bringing a huge crockpot full of chili. I would not let her do any housework, but we had a wonderful visit that day.

Chapter 23

What Now, You Ask?

So, I get my eyes checked every year. I wore glasses, but more importantly, I have diabetes and need to get checked for diabetic retinopathy. Another one of those words, but it's not new to me. I went for my annual eye exam in late January 2025. I was told by my oncologist to make sure the doctor knew I was taking Tamoxifen, as it can cause Glaucoma. I told him. He told me that they do not see that being a problem nearly as much as it used to seem, but he would definitely check for it.

I had noticed a change in my eyesight and thought that it was tied to my A1c score. I have always noticed my eyesight fluctuates as my score goes up and down. During my breast cancer, it got pretty high, and I had seen it coming down. I thought for sure my eyesight was improving with my lowering A1c and that my glasses were now too strong. I told this to my eye doctor, who said we would take a look and find out. We did all the normal tests. He did the puff of air, which always makes me jump, even though I know it is just air. He did the retinopathy exam and the eye exam.

When we were all finished with all of the exams and measurements, he showed me the picture of the back of my eye, showing that there was no diabetic nerve damage. Yes! I worry about this every time. He then went on to tell me that my eyesight had changed, but not for the reason I thought it had. He told me that I had cataracts. He said he could prescribe me new glasses, but that my vision would still be cloudy, and he took out a model of an eye to show me how cataracts affect vision and how surgery works.

We talked about my age. I'm only 56. I'm too young to have cataracts. I asked him what would cause them in someone my age. He said that some of my medications may be the culprit, but that stress can cause it as well. I don't know why he would think I have had stress lately. I later consulted Dr. Google about this. I was curious why I had developed them at my age. I found that fluctuations in A1c scores can also cause cataracts. I have had a lot of fluctuations as I try to navigate controlling my diabetes.

The doctor explained that during cataract surgery, the old, cloudy lens of your eye (which is located in the back of the eyeball, by the way! Who knew?) is removed and a new corrective lens is put in place. I could have my nearsightedness corrected, or I could have my close-up corrected. He said it is a personal preference, but if it were him, he would have his close-up vision correct. Something to ponder.

Fortunately, we have one of the best eye surgery centers in the United States right here in our hometown. I got scheduled there quickly for a consultation and then two surgeries. One for each eye on separate days. So here I am, losing two more days of work. Again, proving how accommodating my employer is.

I chose to correct my nearsightedness and use readers for up close. I really like not having to wear glasses all the time.

Chapter 24
Mid-Life Crisis

For the next part of my story, I need to give you some backstory. In 2016, I was a half-owner in a manufacturing business, and Jim worked there as well. My life was just not where I wanted it to be. I felt stagnant in that job and wanted to do something different. When the opportunity came, I asked my brother to buy out my half. Once the sale was complete, we set a date, and Jim and I walked out for our last time on September 30, 2016. We did not know what we were going to do, but we knew we were going to be alright. He had a number of people asking him to come work for them, and I said I was not too proud to wait tables or check groceries if I had to.

Even though I was not worried and knew something would come along, it was terrifying to leave. We were jumping into the unknown. I had always wanted a tattoo, and I found a Celtic symbol which means "beginnings." About this time, I came across a quote that said, "Trust the magic of new beginnings." That was it. I knew what I wanted.

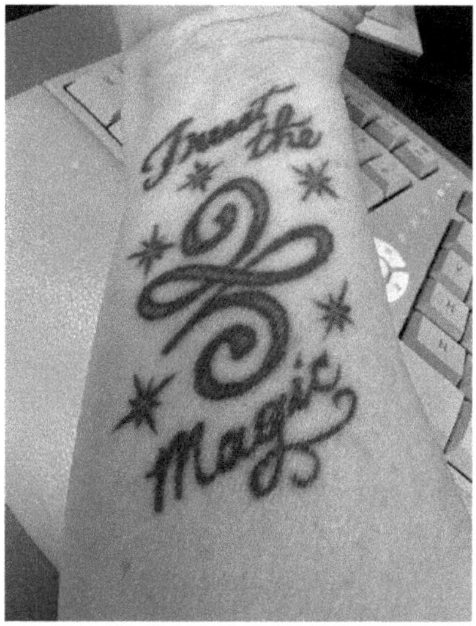

Somewhere around this time, I decided I wanted a handgun. No, I did not plan to shoot anyone. I wanted to have one for protection. I am not left alone often, but we live in the country where there is nobody around to help without a phone call. And going to the range to practice just sounded fun. We shopped and shopped, and I found one I liked and we bought it.

How does all of this tie together, you ask? I called this my mid-life crisis. Buying a sports car, psht! I bought a gun, got a tattoo, and sold my business. How's that for a mid-life crisis?

I called it my temporary retirement. We had the money from the sale of the business to live on while we looked for new jobs. Mine would come, surprisingly, in an accidental encounter at the department store. I was a CASA (Court Appointed Special

Advocate) volunteer for our county program, and I had taken time off from taking cases due to the stress of wanting out of the factory and all that went with it. On New Year's Eve 2016, I literally ran into the executive director, at the time, coming out of the dressing room. The CASA office was short a person in the already small staff, and she wondered if I would be interested in helping out. I started working for the program in January 2017 and worked there until February 2024. I remain a volunteer.

CASA is an amazing program. There is nothing more satisfying than advocating for the best interests of children. I am still a volunteer, but have not worked in the office for over a year now.

I loved working for CASA, but it was a very stressful job and tugged at my heart. I am thankful for my time there and appreciate all that I learned, but I can't imagine having gone through my breast cancer while still working there. I am sure my stress level would have been through the roof.

Chapter 25
Memorialization

So now, you know how my addiction to tattoos began. I have three. But I also want to memorialize this journey. I have been on Pinterest again and talking to Angela and Betsy. I think I have determined I don't need the nipple tattoos, but I do want to have something done to wear as my badge of honor. Angela said her daughter, Victoria, would like to join us as well, and I know Erin will too.

One that I know I want to get is a pink ribbon on the inside of my middle finger. I think I can talk the other girls into it as well.

I have not yet decided what else I want to get or where I want to put it.

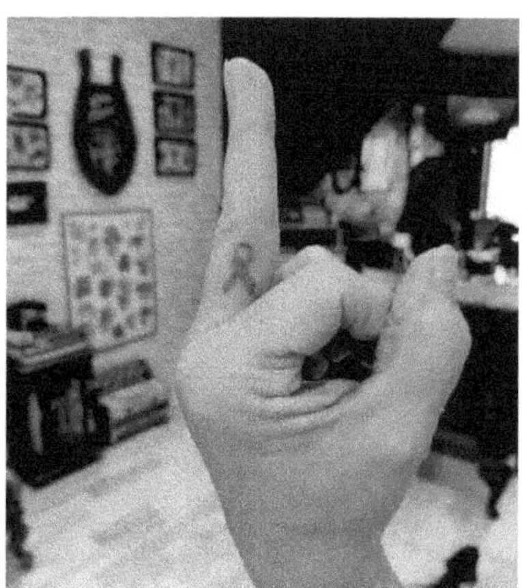

Chapter 26
Feeling Like Me Again

Our children grow up, and we grow older. We change jobs and our parents age. We lose people we love, and life just happens. Somewhere along life's journey, I feel like I lost Me. I stopped wearing make-up or making the effort to look my best. I chose easy hairstyles so I wouldn't have to worry about it.

After my surgery, I decided that since I had these new boobs, I would make an effort. So I started wearing make-up again. I started curling my hair. After my cataract surgery, I no longer needed to wear my glasses, so people began noticing my eyes again and saying they had a twinkle to them.

I have told a few people that I need to lose some weight to show these girls off. I had been seeing the commercials for the new laser liposuction procedures. I thought about asking Dr. Cutie what he thought. But then I decided that I would just try to do it on my own. So far, well… we will get there.

I had someone comment to me the other day that I seemed to be radiating. Maybe I am. I am happier than I have been in a long time. I feel more like myself than I have in years. Plus, I just survived cancer. Why wouldn't I?

Chapter 27

Released

On March 18, we made the trip to Indianapolis for another post-operative appointment. We were told at the February appointment that the Doctor would be present at this one and that if everything looked good, it would be my last visit.

Again, the physician's assistant greeted me and was very pleased with my healing. And for the look of my breasts, there is a space at the top of each one that seems… empty. I call it my divots. We talked about those, and she said that we could possibly do a fat graft at some point if I wanted to. But that was a conversation for another day. She took some pictures and asked me if I would like the before and after photos, and I told her I did not need them.

I was told that I should come in annually to have my implants ultrasound checked for "rupture." She said she does not like that word because they don't actually rupture; they might crack.

Finally, Dr. Cutie came in, took a look, and gave his thumbs up and a fist bump. He told me that I could call him for anything, including the fat graft if I decided I wanted it, anytime between now and when he retires. Have I mentioned he's young? This should give me lots of time to decide if I want to do that.

Before we left, I was told to "Go home and live my life." And that I have.

I came back to work the next day. Everyone knew where I had been the previous day and why. Each time I would tell someone that I had been released with those parting words, I would get a fist bump or a hug. There were even some more tears. And finally, "that sounds like a cause for celebration." I went home and texted our couples' group and asked who wanted to go out that weekend and celebrate. We were able to round up two of the couples and will have the third included at some point. We went out and had a wonderful time. Anytime anybody started to talk about anything negative, we were reminded that we were "celebrating Aimee." And then at the end of the night, one of those sweet couples picked up the bill! Wow, do we have great friends, or what?

And guess what, I am finally crying for myself. Happy tears!

Chapter 28

Life Goes On

The world doesn't stop for you just because you have cancer. During my journey, Jim's dad, who has struggled with a number of health issues, began having some extreme symptoms. His most recent diagnosis was Parkinson's Disease. He was in and out of the hospital and between the hospital and the nursing home for rehabilitation. The last time he was home was before Christmas.

He was treated for the flu during this time, as well as his Parkinson's. My mother-in-law sat with him every day, whether at the hospital or the nursing home. He lost weight and would get to the point that he just would not eat. He would go after his meal with a ravenous hunger but make a face and stop after one or two bites. Having done a little research, I was certain this was a symptom of his Parkinson's, but they continued to treat him for nausea, flu, etc.

This went on longer than I felt like it should, and I finally sat down with Jim's mom and told her that I felt like she needed to accept that Joe was not getting better and was not going to be coming home. She needed to begin making plans for his long-term care. I explained that she needed to tell the staff at the nursing home that he no longer wanted to go to the hospital for anything. She and Jim would meet with the administration to talk about moving him to the long-term care unit of the nursing home. They were advised that we should get a Power of Attorney document so that any of us could make decisions on his behalf. He was able to sign these documents, but more importantly, he was able to sign the DNR document himself. He was clear-minded. His body was just giving up on him.

Eventually, he would lose his voice but would still try to communicate and be positive. One night, I told Jim, "He is tired. He needs our permission to let go." We went in on a Sunday and had our visit with him. We had contacted Erin and Chad to try to come that day. Erin was able to, but Chad was not. When Jim was ready to leave for the day, I told him that I was going to say goodbye to his dad, and then I would leave the room so that he could have some privacy. I told Joe that we understood how tired he was and that it was ok for him to rest. We would all be ok and would take care of one another. I kissed him on the forehead and left the room.

Erin came out to the hallway with me, and I told her that Grandma needed to hear that as much as Grandpa did. We cried together while Jim gave his permission. Jim and I left, and Erin and Justin stayed to say their goodbyes.

Monday morning came, and Jim received a call from his dad's regular nurse letting him know that time was getting short. Jim was able to gather Chad and go back to the nursing home. Chad was able to say his goodbye and went back to work.

Joe passed away on March 10, 2025, with Jim and his mom

at his side. We buried him three days later. We celebrated a very loved man who touched the lives of a lot of local kids whom he had employed over the years. The stories we heard during this time would bring tears and comfort. One of those young men would give the funeral service, and I couldn't have imagined anyone doing a better job.

Life moves on. I am thankful that I was able to get through my storm and provide the emotional support my family needed during this time.

Chapter 29

Parting Thoughts

So that's my story. Eight months. Eight months from diagnosis to release. I survived! I have been told that I have not yet grieved for what I have lost. Maybe that's true, but I don't see it. I have been present and cognizant of what has been going on through this entire journey.

Did I lose my breasts? Yes, I did. But I don't feel it as a loss. Maybe at some point I will, but for now, I view it as a new beginning, without cancer. My reconstructed breasts are not perfect, but they are better than the originals. I used to say they looked at the floor instead of looking forward. You older ladies, or heavier ladies, will understand what I mean by that. My new boobs do not look at the floor. I like that about them. They do still have those divots I talked about earlier, but fat grafting is still an option, and I am considering it more and more. I guess I will have some questions at my one-year appointment. I have struggled to find a bra that pushes my breasts in enough to fill those divots in but remains comfortable and attractive. So far, no Bueno. I am certain once I have lost the weight I want to lose and/or had the fat grafting, I will find what I need and be confident and comfortable.

Speaking of losing the weight I want to lose… I still need to work on my diet, but I have found a workout facility that I love. I have been doing hot/sauna workouts for a while now, and I love them. I highly recommend. I love a good sauna, and working out in one is amazing. I am detoxing and working out. I am exhausted yet exhilarated (don't ask me how, but it's true.)

There is still a level of discomfort in my chest. My implants were placed on top of the muscle due to the size, so I can feel them "pulling." It's not at all painful, just different. They continue to feel heavy. Add to this that I have not fully regained sensation in my breasts. It's hard to explain. I can feel them from the inside, but the skin has no feeling in much of it. I feel like it is "waking up," as Jim puts it. It is just a little disconcerting when I have an itch that I most definitely can feel, because it is coming from the inside, but I cannot feel myself scratching it. Much like when you get a spinal block and can feel a tugging, but cannot feel whatever it is they are doing. It's just weird.

I feel like these are minor inconveniences in the grand scheme of things. I am alive! I did not have to go through Chemotherapy or radiation. I did not have to lose my hair or get sick. I have had a relatively easy time of it. I have been told that I am a warrior, and Jim tells me that I am "tough as hell." I don't feel like I have had to be tough at all. I have been incredibly surprised at the absence of pain through this whole thing. I

Perhaps at some point, I will grieve. But I don't think so. I don't feel as though I have lost anything. OK, I lost a couple of fat bags that were replaced with some perkier artificial fat bags. I lost some time and had to use my vacation for something besides a beachside resort. But I feel like I found so much. I found a family I didn't know I had. I found out how loved I am. I found one-on-one time with Jim and anybody who came to visit. I found strength and patience. I found a new determination to work on making myself better… I found ME.